Facing Breast Cancer

A Guide to Beginning Treatment with Knowledge, Positivity and Support

Hope Suhr

COPYRIGHT

Facing Breast Cancer: A Guide to Beginning Treatment with Knowledge, Positivity and Support

Copyright © 2025 Hope Suhr

TABLE OF CONTENTS

FOREWORD

The day we hear a cancer diagnosis our lives come to a standstill for a short time. It is hard to know where to start after hearing the words our brains don't want to accept, and none of us face the exact same path. Medical words are confusing, diagnostic tests are frightening and treatments are always changing. All the while, the rest of your family and career life goes on as if your mental bandwidth has no limits.

Our best advice is often from people who have already gone through what you are starting to face. The seemingly "simple questions," that you don't want to ask or don't, and now you should ask are already laid out in this wonderful guide on how to manage those tough first steps. Hope Suhr is an incredibly compassionate, thoughtful patient who has gone through the tough times and come out the other side. Her research and organized presentation will provide needed comfort to countless patients that you too will get through this difficult time!

Dr. Kimberly Minesinger

Family Medicine and Hospice & Palliative Medicine

PREFACE

My story, this book, is about more than health battles—it's a testament to resilience, growth, and grace. I willingly share it with others so that they may understand the path my husband and I have walked together—not to seek sympathy, but to ask for patience as I continue to navigate the effects of these past years, as they can be long-lasting, because the process of recovery is ongoing.

Sometimes I may get frustrated, communicate poorly, or make mistakes. I need a little understanding as I carry the weight of personal responsibilities and continue to rebuild.

INTRODUCTION

My Journey with Breast Cancer: A Personal Story of Hope, Resilience, Love, and Recovery

The Discovery

It was January 2021. My husband and I had been spending a lot of time together in our bedroom as he battled his own health issues. We were watching a show one night when, as I leaned over him, I felt something strange—a hard lump on my breast. Daniel, being a physician associate, immediately examined it. He was calm, but I could see the concern in his eyes. Breast cancer runs in my family; my mother is a 25-year survivor, and that legacy weighed heavily on our minds as we prepared to make a doctor's appointment.

We didn't waste any time. Next week, I went in for a mammogram and an ultrasound. I watched the technician's face intently through each test for any hint of what she might be seeing. When she said she'd be back after consulting the doctor, my stomach dropped. Moments later, the doctor came in and calmly explained that we'd need to schedule a biopsy. A million thoughts flooded my mind. One of the scariest was "Crap…I'm here by myself." My thoughts also went to my mom, who is a quadruple cancer survivor, and "what if I have breast cancer? What do I need to do if this is the case?" I was determined to stay calm and take things step-by-step. I don't know how I made it home, but I put on my big girl pants, drove home, and my mind was swimming with the many "what-ifs."

The biopsy confirmed it—I had breast cancer. But the surprising part? It wasn't in the area where we initially felt the lump. Suppose we hadn't noticed that lump, we might not have caught the cancer in its early stages. It was a moment that felt divinely guided; a "God thing," as I like to say. It made me reflect on how life surprises us at a moment's notice; it doesn't always happen at the most opportune time!

The Decision

Within weeks, I met with a general surgeon, then a plastic surgeon, and surgery was quickly scheduled for March 4, 2021. My doctors planned a lumpectomy along with asymmetry surgery to even things out—a reduction from a breast size of 36K to 36G. As nervous as I was, I couldn't help but laugh about this "silver lining." It was time for a much-needed lift—in more ways than one.

The Fight Begins

When we got the post-surgery news, I learned my cancer was at Stage One. We had caught it early, and for that, I was deeply grateful. Still, I had months of treatment ahead: chemotherapy, radiation, and IV Herceptin to tackle any remaining cancer cells. I steeled myself, knowing that these treatments were a necessary part of my journey.

Chemo was tough. My first session felt like an initiation into a club I never wanted to join. The "red devil," as they called it, was particularly brutal. My hair started falling out, and the decision to shave it felt like reclaiming control. It was one of the hardest days, but also a freeing one. I chose a beautiful wig from my stepmom's shop in Newport Beach and braced myself for what lay ahead.

Love and Resilience

Throughout my cancer journey, my husband was my rock. Despite his own struggles, including a below-the-knee amputation on July 22, 2022, he was right by my side. His health journey paralleled mine, and we spent countless hours shuffling between doctors: appointments for him, then for me, and back again for him, and so on and so forth. But we had a system. Fun right? A system to get all our doctor and therapy appointments on the same day so we would get worn out only one or two days. Despite his own disability, he still provided unwavering support, guidance, and research, helping me understand every step.

My family, friends, and neighbors also became an incredible support network. They dropped off groceries and supplies, and shared kind words that lifted my spirits on the hardest days. I must share that even though I received the meals, I still had to prepare the meals and bring them to my husband, and then clean up. It's tough to walk up and down the stairs… it felt like I was climbing Mount Everest. I would make it half way up the stairs and then have to stop. I was exhausted.

I connected with Michelle's Place, a cancer support organization that provided comfort and understanding when I needed it most. It truly felt like an entire village had gathered around us, helping us weather this storm.

Hope Triumphs

July 27, 2022, marked the end of my treatments. I rang the bell at the oncology center with tears in my eyes and hope in my heart. I was a breast cancer survivor! I looked back on everything my husband and I have gone through—the countless doctor visits, treatments, and surgeries. We were battered but not broken. We had faced it all and were still standing, together.

This journey taught me that resilience is built one step at a time. Each small victory, every shared laugh, and every embrace from loved ones became the fabric of my healing. Cancer tested me, tested us, but it couldn't take away our strength, our love, or our faith.

The journey of facing a breast cancer diagnosis can feel overwhelming, especially in the early stages of planning treatment. This guide aims to empower you with essential information, insightful questions for your doctor, and strategies to build a positive support network. Being informed and surrounded by encouraging, understanding people can profoundly affect your experience. Let this book be a gentle guide, offering knowledge, reassurance, and practical advice as you take the first steps in your treatment journey.

Our Journey: Nine Years of Loss, Resilience, Healing, and Growth

I received such great support from my husband, friends, and family.

2014
The journey began with deep loss—my dad passed away on December 27th. The grief was intense, but I pressed forward, needing to stay strong for my family, and sometimes death can bring family chaos. It did! That's another story.

2015
In January, I opened a brick-and-mortar store called Hope's Chest in a new location. The venture was exciting, but family dynamics

brought added stress. As tensions rose, I made the difficult decision to step back from family involvement and focus on my path.

2016

After a year, I closed the store and transitioned to an online-only business—a small but meaningful victory. Around the same time, I entered the insurance industry, a field that offered new opportunities and challenges.

2017

Hallelujah, a free year of total bliss of health!!!!

2018

In October, my husband crushed his foot—a devastating injury with a long recovery. It was the beginning of a series of significant (or profound?) medical issues that would add even more complexity to our lives.

2019

In March, I was diagnosed with skin cancer, melanoma on my back; surgery in July successfully removed it. Just two months later, in May, my husband's foot condition led to the amputation of all his toes. We leaned heavily on each other for strength, undergoing treatments and adjusting to a new normal.

2020

In November, my husband suffered another setback—a secondary infection in his foot required surgery and hospitalization. His recovery was extended and even more challenging.

2021

In January, while focusing on his healing, I discovered I had a lump in my breast and went in right away to get checked. Went to get a mammogram and biopsy. Yup, breast cancer. The diagnosis was a shock, but I knew I had to face it head-on while continuing to care for him and manage my business. March 4th lumpectomy and reconstructive surgery. Then treatment all the way through to July 2022.

2022

February brought another challenge—my husband was diagnosed with 95% arterial blockage and required quadruple open-heart surgery. His operation was scheduled for none other than, yup, March 4th! The same date, one year apart, in the same hospital.

July 22

Daniel opted for a below-the-knee amputation to stop bone remodeling, recurring infections. It was a tough, but necessary decision.

Many months later, the prosthetic was introduced, as healing and shrinking take time. The process of adjusting to prosthetics became a journey of its own, lasting about 15 months.

July 27

I completed my last cancer treatment. Praise God! One week apart. We were in a good place.

CHAPTER 1: Understanding Your Diagnosis

(Clarity, fear, steady ground)
"God is our refuge and strength, a very present help in trouble."
— Psalm 46:1

The first step after a breast cancer diagnosis is understanding what it means. Breast cancer is unique for every individual. Knowing the specific characteristics of your cancer, such as its type, stage, hormone receptor status, and aggressiveness, will help your healthcare team create a tailored treatment plan. Some types of breast cancer grow quickly, while others progress slowly. Treatments vary, and learning about your specific diagnosis is key to understanding why certain treatment paths are recommended over others. Begin by asking your doctor for a clear explanation of your diagnosis and what it means for your health.

You may also have multiple doctors who specialize in different treatments for the different stages of care. Use the below to keep track of this information.

Date of Diagnosis_______________________________________

Doctor's Name_______________________________

Phone Number___________________________________

Specialty____

Address____

Doctor's Name_______________________________
Phone Number_______________________________
Specialty____
Address____

Doctor's Name_______________________________
Phone Number_______________________________
Specialty____
Address____

Doctor's Name_______________________________
Phone Number_______________________________
Specialty____
Address____

Doctor's Name_______________________________
Phone Number_______________________________
Specialty____
Address____

Doctor's Name_______________________________
Phone Number_______________________________
Specialty____
Address____

To best understand your diagnosis and treatment, it is important to know exactly where your cancer is. Use the space below to draw the location of your tumor from a mirror image, noting which breast it is in:

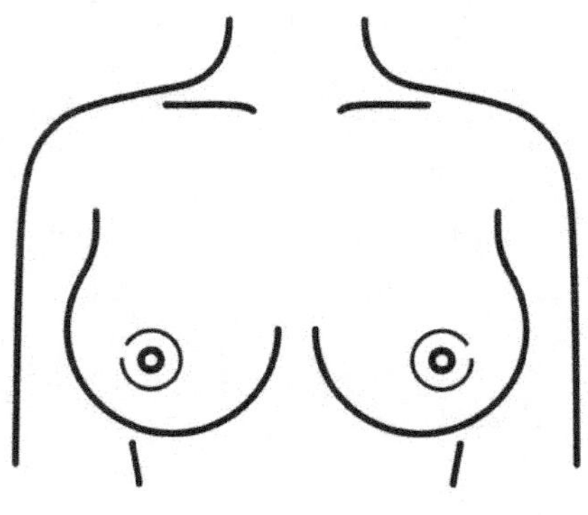

Left   Right

Use this space for important notes, such as "tender to touch," or "area feels hot," or "skin texture is…":

____

____

____

____

____

____

____

____

Embrace hope and support. Beginning breast cancer treatment is undoubtedly challenging, yet having the right information, support, and a positive mindset can make a meaningful difference. Take each step one day at a time, lean on your support network, and trust that you're not alone. This journey is one of resilience, and you have the strength to face each day with hope. Below are questions to ask your doctor about understanding the diagnosis.

Can you explain my specific type of breast cancer and its stage?

What are the characteristics of my tumor?

Is my cancer hormone receptor-positive or HER2-positive? (HER2-positive breast cancer is a breast cancer that tests positive for a protein called human epidermal growth factor receptor 2 (HER2). This protein promotes the growth of cancer cells.)

____

____

____

____

____

BRCA 1&2 Testing: Complete a comprehensive hereditary cancer panel testing, colonoscopy, and DEXA scan, & review results with oncology.

____

____

____

____

____

CHAPTER 2: Exploring Treatment Options

(Wisdom, decision-making, direction)
"Trust in the Lord with all your heart… and He will direct your paths."
— Proverbs 3:5–6

Breast cancer treatment typically involves a combination of options, which might include surgery, chemotherapy, radiation therapy, targeted therapies, and hormonal treatments. Each approach has its purpose, benefits, and potential risks. In some cases, treatment might begin with surgery to remove the tumor, while others may start with chemotherapy to shrink the cancer before surgery. Your doctor will work with you to determine the best sequence and combination of treatments based on the specifics of your diagnosis. Below are examples of key questions to ask your Oncologist. These questions will help establish a strong understanding of your diagnosis, giving you a foundation for the decisions ahead.

What are the treatment plans for my specific type of breast cancer and its stage?

____

____

____

____

____

____

What are the characteristics of my tumor?

____
____
____
____
____

Is my cancer hormone receptor-positive or HER2-positive?

____
____
____
____
____

How aggressive is my cancer, and what does that mean for my treatment?

____
____
____
____
____

Are there additional tests (like genetic testing) that I should consider?

What treatment options do you recommend for me, and why?

What are the goals of each proposed treatment (e.g., surgery, chemotherapy, radiation)?

Is it beneficial for me to start with chemotherapy, surgery, or another treatment?

____

____

____

____

Are there any alternative or emerging treatments I should know about?

____

____

____

____

Will I need a combination of treatments, and if so, in what order?

____

____

____

____

____

Are there any questions I didn't ask, but should have?

____

____

____

____

____

CHAPTER 3: Preparing for Surgery and Procedures

(Surrender, trust, courage)
"Cast all your anxiety on Him because He cares for you."
— 1 Peter 5:7

For many women, surgery is a key component of breast cancer treatment. Your Oncologist and surgeon will work with you to determine whether a lumpectomy, mastectomy, or another procedure is best suited to your situation. In some cases, additional procedures, such as lymph node removal, may be necessary. Your doctor can guide you on what to expect before, during, and after surgery. It's normal to feel anxious, but preparing yourself with information can alleviate some concerns. Below are questions to ask about your surgery.

What are my surgical options, and of those, which do you recommend, and why?

____

____

____

____

____

Will I need lymph node removal?

____

____

____

____

____

How do I limit the risks of lymphedema post op?

____

____

____

____

____

What are some exercises and early treatments for lymphedema?

____

____

____

____

____

Are there options for breast reconstruction, and if so, when would that take place?

____

____

____

____

____

What does recovery from surgery look like?

____

____

____

____

____

What should I know about the risks and benefits of each surgical option?

____

____

____

____

____

CHAPTER 4: Managing Side Effects and Risks

(Strength in weakness, endurance)
"The Lord sustains them on their sickbed."
— Psalm 41:3

Cancer treatments often bring side effects. Understanding the possible effects of chemotherapy, radiation, and other therapies will prepare you to cope and seek the right support. Knowing that side effects are normal and manageable helps reduce fear. Your care team can offer strategies to alleviate them. Below are questions to ask your doctor regarding side effects.

What are the potential side effects of each treatment?

____

____

____

____

____

How can I manage or minimize these side effects?

____

____

____

____

Will my fertility be affected, and if so, are there ways to preserve it?

____

____

____

____

____

What long-term health issues might I face after treatment? For example, vaginal atrophy, pelvic floor dysfunction, osteoporosis, menopause treatment? Is Bio-Identrical HRT an option?

____

____

____

____

____

Are there lifestyle changes that could help reduce side effects, such as diet, exercise, and/or fasting?

____

____

____

____

____

Chapter 5: The Logistics of Treatment

(Order, peace, overwhelm management)
"You will keep in perfect peace those whose minds are steadfast."
— Isaiah 26:3

Breast cancer treatment can be time-intensive, impacting daily routines and responsibilities. Discussing logistics with your care team is essential for planning your life around treatments. This includes understanding your treatment schedule, knowing what to expect in each session, and determining if you'll need support from family or friends to get to and from treatments. Below are questions to ask your doctor regarding treatment logistics.

How long will each treatment take, and what does a typical schedule look like?

____

____

____

____

____

Can I continue working or performing daily activities during
treatment? How much can I push myself?

____

____

____

Where will I receive treatment, and how often will I need to come in?

____

____

____

____

____

Will I need someone to accompany me during treatments?

____

____

____

____

____

What should I bring or prepare for each treatment session?

____

____

____

____

____

Chapter 6: Building a Supportive Circle

(Community, support, connection)
"Carry each other's burdens."— Galatians 6:2

One of the most powerful elements in your journey is the presence of positive, supportive people. Friends, family, and community can lift you up, help you through hard days, and celebrate each step of your progress. Studies have shown that having a strong support system contributes to better outcomes, lower stress, and improved well-being during cancer treatment.

<u>Why Surrounding Yourself with Positivity Matters for Emotional Strength</u>: Supportive people bring encouragement and laughter, helping you stay emotionally resilient. Moreover, it allows you to be your authentic self, which is equally important. Write below the names of people whom you can lean on for positive support. Let them know you are counting on them to help you get through this.

____

____

____

____

____

<u>Reduced Stress</u>: Positive interactions reduce anxiety, which is beneficial for your immune system and overall health. Write below things that make you happy.

____

____

____

____

____

<u>Practical Help</u>: Friends and family can help with transportation, meals, or daily tasks, allowing you to focus on healing. Start a list of friends and family you can put on notice for when you need to go somewhere, or need assistance with preparing meals, or simply need someone to change your sheets on a weekly basis.

____

____

____

____

____

<u>Enhanced Perspective</u>: Supportive loved ones who can remind you of your strengths reinforces hope during challenging times. Prepare a list of your strengths. When you need the support, show it to others and ask them to give you examples of when they thought you were strong.

____

____

____

____

____

<u>Surround yourself with people who make you feel valued, loved, and cared for</u>. Avoid those who may add stress or negativity, as your focus should be on healing and well-being.

____

____

____

____

____

Chapter 7: Seeking Resources and Support

(Provision, help, guidance)
"My God will meet all your needs according to His riches."
— Philippians 4:19

Breast cancer treatment often brings both emotional and financial challenges. Many resources are available to support you, from nutritional counseling to financial assistance. Speak with your care team about accessing these resources. Visit www.clinicaltrials.gov to learn about clinical studies from around the world. Below are questions to ask your doctor about support resources.

Are there support groups and/or resources you can recommend for me and/or my family?

____

____

____

____

Will I have access to a nutritionist, counselor, or other specialists?

____

____

____

____

____

What lifestyle or diet changes would benefit me during treatment?

____

____

____

____

____

Who will be part of my care team, and how do I reach them if I have
questions?

____

____

____

____

____

Are there financial counselors or other resources available to me for
help with the cost of treatment?

____

____

____

____

____

Chapter 8: Planning for Life After Treatment

(Restoration, healing, new season)
"I will restore to you the years that were lost."
— Joel 2:25

Life after breast cancer treatment can bring a mix of relief, anxiety, and adjustment. It's common to have follow-up appointments to monitor health and watch for recurrence. Discuss with your Oncologist what to expect after treatment, including any ongoing lifestyle changes. Below are questions to ask your doctor about life after treatment.

What should I expect in terms of follow-up care?

____

____

____

____

____

Are there signs or symptoms I should watch for?

____

____

____

How can I maintain my health and reduce the risk of recurrence?

Is there a survivorship program available to help me transition post-treatment?

How will we monitor my progress moving forward? Will I need ongoing oncology visits even after remission?

What are my post-treatment surgical options, and what do you recommend?
35

____

____

____

____

____

Chapter 9: The Diet

(Provision, body, care)
"He gives strength to the weary and increases the power of the weak."
— Isaiah 40:29

A balanced diet is crucial for cancer patients as it helps maintain strength, energy, and a strong immune system throughout treatment and recovery. It also aids in managing treatment side effects, reduces the risk of infections, and supports faster healing. A healthy, balanced diet rich in fruits, vegetables, whole grains, lean protein, and healthy fats is generally recommended. While I'm not a qualified dietician, I am qualified to share my biggest health issue. That is the constipation point of this journey - it's real. Prunes became my best friend. Drinking plenty of water is also a vital part of your healing, as it helps rid the body of toxins. Be sure to ask others what helped them (experience is the best knowledge).

Key Food Groups to Focus on:

<u>Fruits and Vegetables</u>: These are packed with vitamins, minerals, and antioxidants, which can help protect cells from damage. Aim for a variety of colors to get a wide range of nutrients.

<u>Whole Grains</u>: Choose options like whole wheat bread, brown rice, and quinoa for fiber and other nutrients.

<u>Lean Protein</u>: Include sources like fish, poultry, eggs, beans, lentils, and nuts to help maintain muscle mass and support overall health.

<u>Healthy Fats</u>: Choose unsaturated fats from sources like avocados, nuts, and olive oil.

<u>Dairy (or plant-based alternatives)</u>: Include dairy products like yogurt or cheese for calcium and protein.

Specific Foods to Consider:

<u>Cruciferous Vegetables</u>: Broccoli, cauliflower, kale, and other cruciferous vegetables are rich in compounds that may have cancer-fighting properties.

<u>Berries</u>: Blueberries, raspberries, and other berries are high in antioxidants.

<u>Antioxidant-rich Fruits and Vegetables</u>: Include colorful options like red peppers, eggplant, and watermelon.

<u>Omega-3 Fatty Acids</u>: Found in fish, flaxseed, and walnuts, Omega-3s may help reduce inflammation and support overall health.

<u>Broths and Soups</u>: These can be easy to digest and provide hydration and nutrients.

<u>Smoothies</u>: A convenient way to consume fruits, vegetables, and protein.

Foods to Limit or Avoid:

<u>High-Fat, Processed Foods</u>: These can contribute to weight gain and may not provide the necessary nutrients.

<u>Sugary Drinks</u>: Limit or avoid sugary drinks and focus on water, tea, or unsweetened beverages.

<u>Excessive Red Meat</u>: While lean protein is important, limit red meat consumption.

<u>Spicy or Acidic Foods</u>: These may irritate the digestive system, especially if you're experiencing nausea or mouth sores.

Important Considerations:

<u>Talk to Your Doctor or a Registered Dietitian</u>: They can provide personalized advice based on your specific cancer type, treatment plan, and individual needs.

<u>Listen to Your Body</u>: Pay attention to how different foods affect you and adjust your diet accordingly.

<u>Stay Hydrated</u>: Drink plenty of fluids, especially water, to help manage side effects like constipation and dehydration.

<u>Eat Smaller, More Frequent Meals</u>: This can be easier on your digestive system if you're experiencing nausea or loss of appetite.

<u>Consider a Build-Up Diet</u>: If you are experiencing weight loss or difficulty getting enough calories, consider adding cream to foods, using butter or oil when cooking, and adding protein to meals.

<u>Exercise</u>: As tolerated as directed by your MD. We are mind body and spirit. Here are some relaxation techniques: journaling, coloring, walking, tai chi, yoga and more.

Medication List

Medication name	Dose	Type (Cap, Tab, Gel, Spray)	Times a Day

EPILOGUE

To the reader, I want you to: listen to your body, get your screenings, and cherish the love that surrounds you. I delayed my mammogram by six months due to COVID—but those screenings are so important. My story is a testament to early detection, faith, and a resilient partnership.

Today, I continue to cherish my family, friends, and every new day with my husband. Life is precious, even in the most difficult of times. We are survivors—grateful, stronger, and filled with hope.

What Michelle's Place and Crystal Rose Mean to me

Michelle's Place has been an invaluable source of information, comfort, and support. I've long been a supporter of this incredible organization and sincerely appreciate the love, care, and compassion they extend to so many. I had the honor of founding the Recycled Bra Art Show in 2012–2013 to help raise funds, and I've volunteered at Michelle's Place Reality Rally fundraiser and participated as a vendor at several events. These groups hold a special place in my heart, and I am forever grateful for all they do.

Thank you to all of you who helped me labor in this book. Janice Leonard, Kimberly Davidson, Traci Wooden, and Daniel Suhr.

ABOUT THE AUTHOR

Introducing Hope Suhr, CEO of Elpis Insurance Services, and your go-to resource for insurance expertise!

With a passion for helping families and businesses, I started to call myself "Hope the Medicare Lady" and have built a reputation for understanding the ins and outs of insurance solutions.

From a young age, I was inspired by my entrepreneurial family and their unwavering work ethic. Now, as a second-generation licensed agent, I continue my legacy by providing custom-tailored policies that ensure the highest level of protection for you and your loved ones.

With my extensive knowledge and access to a wide range of insurance carriers, I can guide you through the maze of health insurance, Medicare, and other insurance options.

But I don't stop there! My commitment extends beyond insurance. My past awards have been recognized as the Inland Empire's Best Lingerie Boutique owner, and I received the SBA Women in Business Champion of the Year Award.

My dedication to empowering others led me to establish the Women's Business Resource Connection, a nonprofit organization supporting local women entrepreneurs.

Everyone needs effective and affordable health insurance. Let us find a plan that fits your lifestyle and budget. You can also find me at in The Medicare Agent Directory at https://medicareagentshub.com/, the American Association for Medicare Supplement Insurance at https://medicaresupp.org/agent/hope/, and on my website at https://elpisinsurance.com/.

Discover the peace of mind of working with a knowledgeable and caring professional. Contact me at (714) 797-9996 for a NO-COST consultation, and let's protect your family and assets together!

#InsuranceExpert #HealthInsurance #Medicare

I'm fully licensed in the State of CA, Lic 0L82681 | State of AZ, Lic18469548 | State of Texas, Tennessee, and other states. I have access to a selection of insurance carriers. Contact me for a NO-COST consultation.

Disclaimer: Hope Suhr is not connected with the Federal Medicare program. I am an independent agent and may contact you. This is a solicitation for insurance.